Top 30 C

Fighting Foods

Diets and Nutritional Meal Plans to Manage, Overcome, and Prevent Cancer

By

Kim Hilton

Top 30 Cancer-Fighting Foods

First edition. June, 2018.

Copyright © 2018 Kim Hilton

Written by Kim Hilton

Books by The Same Author

- Boost Your Energy Levels: 60 Natural Ways to Get Rid of Fatigue, Dizziness, Weakness, And Lack of Motivation

- How to Get Rid Of Stretch Marks Naturally

- How to Break Sugar Cravings with Nutritional Supplements: Healthy and Natural Alternatives

- The Anti-Anxiety Cookbook: Nutritional Plan to Cure Depression and Anxiety (Stress Relief and Mental Health Cookpot)

- Eating Disorder Recovery Workbook: How to Recover from

Eating Disorder On Your Own (Anorexia, Bulimia Nervosa, And Binge Eating)

-
-
-
-

- Natural Treatments for Yeast Infection: How to Cure a Yeast Infection Using Home Remedies

Table of Contents

Introduction

"Cancer is caused by an unregulated growth of abnormal cells in the body. With many causes, there are over two hundred types of cancers."

Major causes of cancers include hereditary and faulty genes, radiation, exposure to harmful chemicals and toxins, obesity, smoking, pathogens and microbes, chronic stress (causes hormonal problems which can cause cancer), chronic inflammation, some drugs and vaccines, emotional problems,

bad water, and lastly unhealthy foods.

How Bad Foods Cause Cancer

The type of foods you eat can either cause cancer or cure it; regular intake of unhealthy and junk foods is the leading cause of cancer worldwide, not hereditary or other causes.

This is because nutrition plays an important role in your life. Your body uses nutrients gotten from foods to build and repair damaged tissue parts. It also uses these nutrients to produce new cells. Ultimately, when the building material is faulty you don't expect the building to be strong.

Unhealthy and empty-calorie foods commonly called junks suppress the immune system and make the body susceptible to cancer and other diseases. When you eat healthy foods, you boost your immune system and you build your body with quality material and not junks.

Some bad foods that both cause cancer and raise the risk of cancer are:

• Refined sugar and sugary foods and drinks; this is the biggest cause of cancer, sugar in all its names and forms like aspartame, high-fructose corn syrup, mono-sodium glutamate, and the rest artificial sweeteners feed cancer cells.

They also cause a sharp rise in the levels of insulin thereby disrupting the levels of the hormone; diabetes medications are being used to fight cancer cells showing the correlation between cancer cells and sugar.

Avoid refined sugar in all forms; they increase the multiplication of cancer cells, go for natural alternatives like raw honey, maple syrup, stevia, or coconut sugar.

• Genetically modified foods cause cancers and tumors in those who eat them regularly; they contain unnatural substances and even viruses and other microbes in most cases that cause cancer.

• Farmed fish are treated with hormones, antibiotics, pesticides, unhealthy feeds and other carcinogens and they are lacking in omega-3 fatty acids.

- Grilled red meat, most especially hot dogs release carcinogenic amines. The process of grilling changes the molecular and chemical of the meat and lead to the release of heterocyclic aromatic amines.

Better alternatives of meat preparation are boiling, baking or preparing it on a skillet.

- Excessive consumption of alcohol causes cancer.

- Hydrogenated oils and Trans-fats are extracted from their source through a chemical process and more chemicals are also used in the production to improve the appearance and taste, all these damage the cell membrane structure and cause cancer.

• Conventional dairy and dairy products reduce the levels of the hormone 1,25-dihydroxyvitamin D3, this hormone protects men from cancer of the prostate.

• Microwaved foods are not healthy either and they both increase the risk of cancer and cause cancer by the process of radiation; microwaved popcorn is the largest cause of lung cancer next to smoking.

•	Smoked foods, salted and pickled foods: they are dense with nitrates which preserve the foods and extend the shelf-life. Regular intake of these foods lead to the accumulation of nitrates in the body, this toxic compound causes havoc at the cellular level and leads to cancer.

Pickled foods exclude fermented foods made at home.

• Processed and canned foods are filled with additives, colorants, artificial sweeteners, artificial flavors and the container they are packed in are lined with Bisphenol-A (BPA) which is a carcinogen.

Plastic cans, water lines, and thermal papers all contain BPA. Avoiding canned and processed foods protect your body from cancer.

• Soda and carbonated drinks.

According to the official report on study about unhealthy foods consumed by

Americans: "These drinks are loaded with sugars of all kinds, dyes, artificial flavors, high-fructose corn syrup, and other additives that are dangerous to the body."

Consuming drinks labeled "diet" contains aspartame which acts as rat poison to the human cells.

• Refined white flour has been robbed of all its nutrients and fibers. It raises the levels of insulin in the body without offering any nutrient, excess intake of products made with refined white flours leads to insulin resistance and this raises the risks of development of cancer.

These foods listed above have been implicated as the causes of cancer, the best way to prevent and fight off cancer is to eat healthy foods, make sure they are organic and this should also include lots of fruits, vegetables and herbs.

Top Thirty Cancer Fighting Foods

1. Dark Green Leafy Vegetables

Dark Green Leafy Vegetables are saturated with powerful antioxidants and phytochemicals that help in the reversal of cancer and cancer related ailments. These include beta-carotene, and isothiocyanates, they fight cancer and detoxify the body at the cellular level. They stop the division of cancer cells.

Don't overcook them, cook them lightly and you should also try to juice them or make smoothies with them.

2. Cruciferous Vegetables

These included cabbage, broccoli, Brussels sprouts, cauliflower, and others are glutathione, the most powerful antioxidant in the body. It expels free radicals which causes cancer from all nooks and crannies of the body.

They also contain isothiocyanates, indoles and sulforaphanes, these compounds protect the DNA and body cells, they prevent cancer and activate detoxifying enzymes.

3. Probiotics

These are friendly bacteria that boost the immune system and fight off cancer. Fermented foods and cultured organic dairy and products are rich sources of probiotics.

4. Green Tea

Green tea stops the spread (metastasis) of cancer, it slows the progression and puts a halt to the rapid division of abnormal cells.

5. Raw Garlic

This herb heals cancer and scavenges free radicals from the body.

6. Carrots

This is a rich source of beta-carotene, falcarindiol, and falcarinol which fights cancer and aid detoxification.

7. Onions

Onions are rich in powerful compounds that fight the formation of nitrosamines and other carcinogens in the body.

8. Apples

They contain procyanidins, this compound kills cancer cells and it prevents cancers in the digestive system like colon cancer.

9. Bran Cereal

They are very rich in fibers which prevent colon cancer and cancer causes by obesity. These fibers are also foods for the friendly bacteria in the gut.

10. Health Virgin Oils

Unrefined healthy oils like coconut oil, olive oil, flaxseed oil, cod liver oil, almond, jojoba, Neem and many others including essential oils fight and prevent cancer and they are better alternatives to these unhealthy refined oils.

11. Artichoke

This herb contains silymarin, a strong antioxidant that fights cancer. It is used in the treatment of skin cancer.

12. Ginger

This is strong herb that fights all types of cancer. Take ginger tea as much as you can daily and try to use fresh ginger roots.

13. Peas

These legumes contain a rich amount of coumestrol, a phytochemical similar to estrogen that helps in fighting cancer especially stomach cancer.

14. Peppers

Chili peppers, black peppers, ball peppers, yellow peppers and red peppers all contain powerful cancer fighting properties. Add then generously to your meals.

15. Seaweed

This herb is loaded with many anti-carcinogenic compounds. It contains fucoidan, a complex polysaccharide which makes cancer cells self-destruct.

16. Dark Chocolate

70% dark chocolate is rich in polyphenols, proanthocyanidins and many other antioxidants that fight cancer. A square of dark chocolate has twice the same effects as taking many glasses of red wine.

16. Orange-coloured Fruits and Vegetables

The pigments responsible for the colour of fruits and veggies are powerful phytochemicals that help the body prevent and fight cancer. You should eat lots of sweet potatoes, squash, citrus fruits, pumpkins, berries and other colourful plants.

17. Eggs

Eggs are dense in vitamin D; this fortifies the immune system and increase the population of white blood cells. Also expose yourself to minimum sunlight at least thirty minutes daily.

18. Beets

They contain betalain, a powerful antioxidant that fights cancer. They induce the apoptosis of cancer cells and halt metastasis.

19. Pomegranate

Unsweetened pomegranate juice raises the levels of antigens in the body and help fight cancer.

20. Grapefruit

Pink and red grapefruits are rich in lycopene which is a potent anti-cancer nutrient.

21. Dates

This sweet fruit is rich in polyphenols than any fruits or vegetables. They fight cancers caused by oxidation and free radicals.

22. Avocado

This fruit is loaded with mono-unsaturated fats that aid the body absorb antioxidants from foods.

23. Mushrooms

These are strong immune enhancers and they fight cancer. Reishi, maitake and Cordyceps are commonly used mushrooms in the treatment of cancer.

24. Grapes

Red grapes have powerful antioxidants that fight against different types of cancer.

25. Beans

Navy beans and black beans are powerful foods that fight cancer.

26. Cooked Tomatoes

Heat activates lycopene, a powerful antioxidant and strong cancer fighter.

27. Wild-caught Fish

Wild-caught are dense in anti-inflammatory compounds and omega-3 fatty acids which help fight off cancer.

28. Nuts and Seeds

These are dense in powerful phytonutrients and omega-3 fatty acids and they include sesame seeds, flaxseeds, hemps seeds, chai seeds, sunflower seeds, pumpkin seeds, walnuts, almonds and Brazil nuts.

29. Turmeric

The active compound Curcumin one of the most powerful anti-cancer foods; it stops the flow of blood to cancer and tumor cells and shrinks their sizes. Take turmeric with black pepper to boost the absorption of curcumin.

30. Berries

Almost all berries have a high content of antioxidants. These include strawberries, blueberries, cherries, raspberries, blackberries, camu camu and goji berries.

They are rich in vitamin C, gallic acid, proanthocyanidins antioxidants, phenols, zeaxanthine, cryptoxanthin, lycopene, polysaccharides and lutein which all help in healing cancer and enhancing your immunity.

Books by The Same Author

- <u>Boost Your Energy Levels:</u> 60 Natural Ways to Get Rid of Fatigue, Dizziness, Weakness, And Lack of Motivation

- <u>How to Get Rid Of Stretch Marks Naturally</u>

- <u>How to Break Sugar Cravings with Nutritional Supplements:</u> Healthy and Natural Alternatives

- <u>The Anti-Anxiety Cookbook:</u> Nutritional Plan to Cure Depression and Anxiety (Stress Relief and Mental Health Cookpot)

- Eating Disorder Recovery Workbook: How to Recover from Eating Disorder On Your Own (Anorexia, Bulimia Nervosa, And Binge Eating)
- 100 Health Hacks Nobody Ever Told You: Natural Tips and Tricks for Enhanced and Prudent Well-Being
- How to Lower Blood Pressure Naturally & Quickly: Powerful Tricks to Deal with Hypertension Using Supplements and Other Natural Remedies
- Reverse Type 2 Diabetes: How to Control and Prevent Diabetes Naturally

- Urinary Tract Infection Treatment: Home Remedies for Urinary Tract Infections and Prevention Methods
- Natural Treatments for Yeast Infection: How to Cure a Yeast Infection Using Home Remedies

36631305R00023

Printed in Great Britain
by Amazon